What real w... are saying about
STUFF YOUR (SUPER) MOM FORGOT TO TELL YOU...

Prologue

It's amazing to think you were carefully listening to me and watching me and remembering what I said all those years ago. My memories of our exchanges may be a bit different than yours, but the end result created a beautiful, confident, and independent woman. Your (super) mom is so proud of her (super) daughter! Congrats on your first of many books.
Susie, 64, Super-Mom of the Author

Step 1: Become a Full-time Model

This is the behind the scenes inspirational talk us gallant women long for as we prepare for the runway of life. So, cue fierce theme music, dim the lights, spotlight on me, I am undeniably ready to strut my confidence, my flaws, my sexy, my strength, my uniqueness, my sincerity, and my power.
But first I need to embrace my signature walk...
Ashley, 34, Super-Model to Everyone

Step 2: If you're not Horny, Break-up!

This chapter perfectly sums up the most pivotal relationship of my life. It was the one in which I realized that valuing myself means so much more than the fleeting value another person can offer me. The awareness of this taught me how to truly love myself enough to never feel the need to sacrifice my values for the sake of feeling important to someone other than me.
Kendra, 39, Balance Goddess

Step 3: Own your O

I love the term MET, as that describes what orgasms have been to me: metaphysical energetic transformation. I discovered my first MET in a lucid dream around the age of nine, and I never looked back, seeking again and again the transcendence that masturbation brought. I have used masturbation to calm myself, find myself, discover myself, and, I'd add, over the years, to know, for certain, that MET comes from my physical, emotional, mental and spiritual alignment as well.
Jessie, 52, Gently Fierce Expander

Step 4: So Long, Ms. Humility

Sometimes we apologize not because we don't re-

alize our worth, but because we feel like we're not allowed to show it. But it's better to be a jerk occasionally than sorry constantly. You can revel in your successes, they're yours to revel in. #sorrynotsorry"
Fatima, 21, Purveyor of Truths

Step 5: Blow Some Shit UP!

I am finally 42, with a reasonably healthy self-concept- so why am I still stuck? Fear and judgment have somehow invaded my mind. Like the Death Star, it is time to blow it to pieces.
I enjoyed this chapter because it gave me the opportunity to take the self-inventory and re-establish my goals. Talking to my son also helped me see that my career is important and valuable.
Andrea, 42, Counselor to Dreamers

Step 6: Get Married (or not)

As a young girl, I was never planning a wedding or coming up with names for my future offspring. As I got older I still never felt that urge to "settle down." I began to feel awkward and uncomfortable when people asked "When do you think you will get married?" Amy validates my inner need for independence and my desire to wait for the right

kind of partner to come into my life. Thank you for cheering for women to be more in control of this aspect of adulthood!
Heather, 42, Education Goddess

Step 7: Have Children (or not)

Amy points out societal and family expectation sign-posts on the drive towards our unique destiny. She shows we can conceive who and what to take for the ride...and shows where and when we can just get off.
Kristin, 35, Soul Whisperer

Step 8: Make Your Escape Plan

After reading this chapter I have been motivated to make a few escapes from my regular routine. The first escape is to the gym. This place causes me much anxiety but once there and I work out I feel so much better. Another escape will be to dance class. I want to learn to line dance so that when I go to events I can be on the floor enjoying myself and not sitting on the sidelines watching the world. And my final escape would be to a yoga class; a regular, beginner's class. My first experience with yoga was to Bikram Yoga which as wayyyyyyy out of my comfort zone- but because I was with friends I felt safe enough to try it. I enjoyed it but know that

it is not for me. I love the feeling of yoga and would love to take the chance to escape to it again.
Erica, 46, Family Peace Guru

Step 9: Your Stress Ain't Cute

When I read "Your Stress Ain't Cute" I could see myself all over the descriptions on the pages. As Amy described draining situations, I could see the same situations in my life, and how I was unconsciously prioritizing them over my happiness. I feel like I was given permission to not be frazzled, and to be in charge of how I want to live. When I listed the 5 things I wished I didn't have to do at the end of the chapter, it was an eye opening reflective experience that gave me clarity to make changes to lower stress in my life.
Carrington, 29, Mom-preneur with the Power to Detox Anything

Step 10: Meditate or Die

Meditate or die sounds extreme doesn't it? Whelp after reading this chapter and working with the author I have come to the conclusion that meditation is truly an act of self-love. Some may interpret this as being selfish and I am totally fine with that assessment. Through meditation I have begun to realize that I am the most important person in my life; I cannot muster up the energy to take care of my parents, partner or friends if I have not taken time for myself. Without meditation, I find that I am short-tempered, moody, and prefer isolation when I lose my soul connection – I literally feel myself wilting.

The practice of meditation teaches me to be grateful, compassionate, and appreciative of my life even when it's difficult. It stokes my quiet fire of courage and helps to quell my anxieties and fear.

Remember… meditation saves lives – not just your life, but the others around you!

Ashanti, 37, Advocate of the Selfish!

Step 11: Help Yourself to Happiness

Giving back has always been important to me, but I felt guilty that some volunteer opportunities seemed draining or awkward. In this chapter, Amy helps us to consider the idea that it's ok to serve in ways that you find truly fulfilling. Now, I feel free to use my gifts in my own unique way for the good of others.

Rachel- 31, Joyful Business-mom

Step 12: Find a Sister-Wife

There's a quote from Jurassic Park that fits so well with this chapter. It says something to the ef-

fect of, "Just because we CAN, doesn't mean we SHOULD." We can try to do it all by ourselves, but learning to live, give, and take together is really the way to go. Thanks for the reminder!
Elizabeth, 35, Full-time Adventure Seeker

Step 13: Choose Your Tribe

No having the benefit of a fantastic family structure I appreciate the advice to make my own tribe. Amy's advice in this chapter speaks to many of us who replace a sub-standard family with stellar friends. In addition, Amy is so super-dooper cool and I can't believe she wrote a whole, big, giant book!
Susan, 45, Cerebral Champion for Questioners

STUFF YOUR (SUPER) MOM FORGOT TO TELL YOU...

about orgasms, apologizing, meditation, and more

13 Steps to Activate Your Super Powers

By Amy Brooks

© Amy Brooks 2015

To all the women in my family who have come before me, thank you for living bigger than folks expected. You showed me my potential just by living out yours.

Life is short, but shouldn't be small.

TABLE OF CONTENTS

Prologue i
Preface.. 1
Step 1: Become a Full-time Model 9
Step 2: If You're Not Horny- Break-up!! 19
Step 3: Own Your O 29
Step 4: So Long, Ms. Humility 39
Step 5: Blow Some Shit Up! 53
Step 6: Get Married…or Not 65
Step 7: Have Kids…or Not 75
Step 8: Make Your Escape Plan 85
Step 9: Your Stress Ain't Cute 93
Step 10: Meditate or Die 105
Step 11: Help Yourself to Happiness 119
Step 12: Find a Sister Wife 129
Step 13: Choose Your Tribe 139
The (Super) People Who Made This Book Possible 147
About the Author 151

PREFACE

❖

Having a mother like Susie means you don't have to figure things out all alone. You don't have to ask friends or look online (although that wasn't really an option for me growing up in the 80's). My mother didn't hesitate to answer questions or point out areas of disagreement. To this day, she is still quick to chime in with information and advice for her four grown-ass children. Being raised in such a communicative family meant you had to be careful what you asked, or at least be ready for the answer you were going to get.

During the first "no holds barred" discussions logged in my memory, I can distinctly recall sitting in the passenger seat of our blue Honda when I was in 3rd grade. From what I can remember, I turned to my mom who was sitting in the driver's seat, and asked her how humping made babies. Earlier that day I had witnessed a conversation between the twin boys who lived across the street from us that referenced this subject with giggling and knowing glances. They were joking about someone "humping" someone else. I hated that I had absolutely no idea what that meant. I knew they thought it was funny, but their statement didn't provide much by way of context clues. Was it like tickling? Were they hitting each other? Was it like thumping someone, but maybe gently?

My mother put the car in park, took the key out of the ignition, and turned her body so that she faced me. Oh no. What did I just ask? This looked serious. She proceeded to stick out her index finger on her right hand and make a circle with her left hand. What could this possibly have to do with humping, I thought frantically.

"Amy, a man has a penis and a woman has a vagina. What the boys were talking about had to do with sex. That's when a man puts his penis inside a woman's vagina," she said while inserting her right finger into the circle of her left hand. AHHHHHHHH!

This talk is representative of so many open conversations we had throughout my youth. My mother's background in early childhood education was one contributing factor, but I also think a major reason why she was always so forthcoming was because she wanted us to come to her for information. By tackling sensitive issues proactively, she could tell us about sex and pregnancy in a way that aligned with our morals. We didn't need to wait until our school told us generic information in Health class; we already had the scoop from our one-one-one chats at home. She was an open book and was candid when addressing any topic we asked her about.

That being said, my mother didn't always wait for a specific question to give us her thoughts. I learned about fellatio when I exclaimed, "this sucks" while looking at something unappealing she was preparing for dinner.

"Amy, don't say 'sucks' that implies something sexual. It means…"

Or the time during my college years when we were driving to my aunt and uncle's house and she turned to me and said, "I hope you know that if you or any of your friends get pregnant, we would want you to keep the baby. Daddy and I will raise it as our own till you're older. It wouldn't be easy, but it's the right thing to do."

"Okay, mom….uggh," I would invariably reply. I didn't love these conversations, but I definitely remember them to this day.

Beyond all the real talk, my mom also modeled all the behaviors the feminist movement encouraged; she made her own choices to ensure her own happiness. For starters, my mother married an awesome man who supported her every move. I witnessed my mom work full-time, then part-time, become a stay-at-home caretaker, build a business out of our home (Brehm's Baskets!), and then return to her career as a teacher. She empowered my father to be our primary parent in her absence and shared household duties with him. She showed me as mothers, it's important that we actually *allow* our spouses to be co-parents: to make child-rearing decisions, spend time independently playing with children, and to take care of their basic needs. It's not easy to let go of some of these aspects of parenting, especially since our spouses will do things differently than we often prefer.

My father, as many fathers do, demonstrated the qualities that I looked later for in a spouse.

My parents' marriage and co-parenting has been a blueprint for my current reality as a wife to a smart, funny, hard-working man and in my role as the mother of three very active little boys.

* * *

This is a book is for all of my friends and acquaintances who have shared stories with me about what they discussed (or didn't discuss) with their mothers growing up. This is a book for women who may have forgotten the wise teachings of their mothers or weren't paying enough attention the first time around. This is an opportunity for us to reflect on aspects of our lives that fuel us: our desires, our expectations, and even our frustrations.

Talking about our role as a "model" for other women and girls, our ability to refrain from apologizing habitually, actually enjoying sex with an orgasm (or five), finding peace with our marital and reproductive choices, and taking time for exploration and relaxation is essential. As the years between the feminist movement and today continue to grow, we need to reevaluate what we want out of our lives. Do we want the high-pressure job? Are we really interested in getting married and having kids? What options do we have to deal with stress? Finally, who do we turn to for support and personal growth?

Let's start the conversation within this safe space. I'm not going to pull the car over and make eye-contact while I tell you about the role of the penis and the vagina, but you will read some concepts that affirm your convictions and some ideas that test your boundaries. Either way, I hope that each chapter allows you to gain clarity about what you want in your life. Through reading, reflection, and possibly discussion with other women, you can define your desires, set clear expectations, and work through some of your frustrations.

It's time.

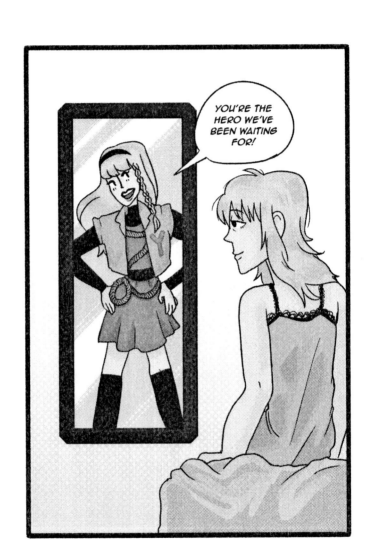

STEP 1

❖

BECOME A FULL-TIME MODEL

In addition to writing this fem-focused book, I work with cool kids every Monday through Friday to improve their communication skills, research ability, love of literature, word choice, and public speaking. Yes, friends, I am an English teacher.

Working with middle school and high school students has cracked me open to so many things. The #1 lesson I've learned is that regardless of our age, we can all learn more about ourselves and grow. If you're open to the lessons around you, your life choices and your interactions with others will show you exactly who you are. You'll also see your influence on the world…and how you're a model for others.

In my lifetime, I've seen my students reflect back whatever I was dishing out. I have watched anti-readers fall in love with *Antigone*. Teens who think they hated rhetoric have become obsessed with ethos, pathos, and logos once they see how it can improve their speech on gay rights. Their excitement didn't blossom in spite of my presence, it existed *because* of my example. When I get all passionate about their poetry or use of polysyllabic words, they giggle and give me more. They also love it (and tease me) when I cry over their autobiographical writing. In essence, we are a room full of energy-sharing souls. It's pretty great.

Kids are brilliant at recognizing authenticity, so I understand it's up to me to bring my full-self to the planning of every lesson. I have seen the greatest success when my "best-me" shows up. When I stay present and focused on the positives, dynamic stuff happens.

We can also learn a few things about ourselves, and how we influence others, when we reflect on our personality. If you're not sure what I mean, start noticing the behaviors that are being reflected back to you. Become sensitive to the energy exchange you have with others. Figure out how your actions are causing reactions and tweak as necessary. As a "model" for others, it's important to be honest with yourself. We all have super powers *and* emotional hang-ups.

I'm ready to admit that I am a hyper, loving, forgiving, impatient woman. I enjoy debate, but hate being interrupted. I adore young people, but find their constant need for guidance exhausting. I want to be needed, but I cannot give away all of myself. I put myself first in many ways that others probably would consider selfish. My temper often flairs up when I'm hungry, tired, or over-stimulated. Yeesh, I sound like a newborn.

I like being happy and positive, but it's a moment-to-moment struggle some days. We have three manic boys who demand all of me. They expect me to be truly present when I come home after a full day with hormonal, angsty teens. They watch how I am as a mom and how I balance my career with my role as one of their caretakers. They observe me living life in a big, bold way as a woman in a household of males. They also see me at my worst when I feel too tired to be patient or even kind.

I'm still growing and my three boys give me constant feedback along the way. They tell me if I'm being unfair with treatment, if I promised something that I seem to be neglecting, or if I need to give them more hugs and kisses. Children are often the mirrors we need if we want to grow. They can call bullshit without saying a word because they are *always* watching or ear-hustling everything around them. Ultimately, they mirror us in their words and actions. Once a child repeats something you've said, it's hard to deny your impact. Watching my oldest son lose his temper is like watching a reenactment of my own meltdowns. I have recently learned to accept how much my boys learn to receive love and react to stress by watching me; they mimic my responses in every way. Sigh.

The idea that kids watch you may seem simplistic, but it holds a very important lesson: The first step to becoming a confident woman is to OWN YOUR POWER. You *are* a model and others *are* watching you whether you like it or not. Your negative body language, flirtations with men, name-calling of women, complaining about your job, and your philosophy on food are being observed at all times. You and I wish our children, and any other human we interact with, would only think of us on our best, most polished, days. In an ideal scenario, their impressions of us would feel similar to uplifting Facebook videos, look as polished as an Instragram photo, and sound as clever as a Twitter post. Instead, we are being watched even when we're tired, grumpy, and bra-less.

Alas, you're projecting you-ness at all times so you should consider the messaging you're sharing with the world. Your goal is not to be perfect, serene, flawless, or any other state of (impossible) being. It is understood that we are all striving for balance, but the purpose of this first chapter is to establish that, for better or worse, we are being watched. Therefore, by improving yourself, your outlook, and your life choices you will only positively impact everyone you know. No biggy.

For now we are going to start with increasing your level of authenticity. I want you to start living as 100% you. Model for others what it means to be really you, unique and quirky and fun.

"Ohhhh, authenticity is easy," you say. I would challenge that most women do *not* live authentically. Instead we subconsciously conform to societal expectations that we outwardly reject. I'm now going to repeat that Women's Studies approved sentiment for effect: We all know what choices or actions we *should* take to live authentically, but most of us choose to stay within the confines society has put on us as women. We are still spending too much time worried about pleasing others through our behavior and our appearance and even apologizing for our strong opinions and voice. We prioritize the needs of others over our own and we value being helpful over being heard. Unfortunately, most of the time we keep ourselves in check without much outside enforcement.

This book is meant to be a step in a new direction, but it will ask you to think about the limits that you have put on yourself through the years. I don't say that lightly. When someone implies that you have limiting beliefs about yourself; and, therefore, limiting beliefs about other women, it's natural to feel defensive. But let's also recognize that we get lots of mixed messages. Many of our skewed perceptions about living life as a confident woman come from decades of watching other female "models." Since we are all contributing members, we all have a responsibility to consider.

So you're a model. Deal with it. Strut your stuff! Don't tell yourself the lie that you can live your life without affecting others. Don't deny the role you play in every other female's existence. When you go to graduate school, achieve greatness in your field, win an award, uplift your sisters, or speak truth to sexism, we all share in that energy. It feels great!

On the other hand, please do us the courtesy of also acknowledging that when you degrade a fellow female, act powerless at work or at home, tell others that you're too fat for love, or encourage a young lady to chose a more "reasonable" dream for herself, we also share in that energy.

We all share in that energy.

You are a model.

You are the model.

You are the model we all need to learn from.

We need confident, whole, beautiful women to show us how it's done.

You are the hero we've been waiting for.

You are the model everyone is watching.

Step 1: Become a Full-Time Model

Let's Get Reflective...

1. **How would you describe your personality?**

   _____

   _____

   _____

   _____

   _____

2. **What women do you consider models in your life? Describe their influence.**

   _____

   _____

   _____

   _____

   _____

3. Who is "watching you" on a daily basis?

4. When have you noticed your energy or behavior reflected back to you?

5. What are two things that you do on a regular basis that don't reflect your authentic self? In other words, what are two things you do that are less about what you *want* and more about what you're *supposed to do*?

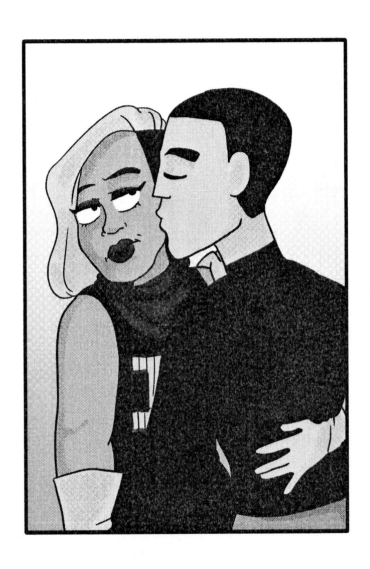

STEP 2

❖

IF YOU'RE NOT HORNY- BREAK-UP!!

Romantic love is a goal to which many women (and men) aspire. It is a place of warm acceptance spiked with sexual abandon. If you find yourself craving companionship without sexual expression, then I would like to suggest that "friendship" may be a better term to define your relationship. In general, "romantic" love is charged with sensual energy that takes the bond between two people to a higher vibration and a more intimate level. The attraction that we crave comes from the sacral chakra and is based on an energy exchange that is rarely given the respect it deserves. Luther Vandross' songs, E.E. Cummings' poems, and Nicholas Sparks' novels do a decent job of transporting us to the place of pseudo-romantic bliss, but until you have found your libido intertwined with someone else's, there is no way of knowing the magic that is love.

Before you worry that I'm describing lust or the physical attraction that can blossom during a spontaneous interaction with someone you think is handsome or beautiful, don't fret. I would like to argue that everything in paragraph one could describe an aging marriage like mine, which is already 16 years old. I'm happy to say I'm still super hot for my honey. I'd also argue that romantic love doesn't explode and dissipate; it is a slow simmer that bubbles up on a regular basis. After you spark the love, you protect the heat, and over time you stoke the flames in order to maintain the long-term lusty feelings.

If you would like romantic love and you want to stay in a state of continued attraction with your partner, you have to set your standards pretty high. In order to achieve this, you need to demand a certain level of horny-ness at the beginning of your relationship. Through the years, I have noted that my female counterparts sometimes justify staying with someone they find appealing and pleasant even if they don't seem particularly turned on by that "special" someone.

If you don't feel aroused by your boyfriend/girlfriend after two months of dating, you need to question the trajectory of your relationship. This is where the high standards come in; when you establish non-negotiable rules for yourself, you can stick to your standards. My romance rule: when I was on the dating scene I always broke up with a guy I was dating once I didn't want to kiss him anymore. I am very anti-pity kissing. Even if things are going really well in regard to our scheduled activities and friendly banter, as soon as I realized the kapow(!) factor was not happening with the kissing, I broke it off.

For the record: lips pushing against lips is not inherently a pleasant physical activity. If a random person pushed his lips on yours, you would not be pleased. We all acknowledge that kissing, especially mouth-kissing, is extremely intimate and potentially mind-blowing. So why would you continue pushing your lips against someone else's lips if it wasn't pleasurable? This logic made sense to me when I was dating and I realized that when I was tuned into my physical/emotional response to kissing, it was a *very* early indicator of my soul connection to the other person. If my soul wasn't "feeling it," it sent me the message to move on. It was my job to listen.

Through conversations and observations, I have learned that many folks don't move on; they stay in relationships, even early on, because they hope it will get better. Or, possibly worse, they stay because it's not really "that bad." Not that bad?! You deserve an outstanding lover and partner. I'd like to invite you to make lots of male and female friends. Enjoy your work colleagues, church acquaintances, and neighborhood busybodies, but DO NOT tether yourself to another flesh-encapsulated spirit unless they meet your standards!

This is super-important because women are sensitive; we need to make sure we don't smother this natural gift with complacency. If we take step after step down the path of lowered expectations, we eventually round the corner and find ourselves in Mediocre City. You do not want to live your life in Mediocre City! You do not want things to be average. You, beautiful goddess, deserve greatness.

A friendly reminder, your partner deserves greatness as well. You are a collaborator with your dating partner and together you are co-creating the reality you'll end up with. If they are not willing to verbalize the mismatched energies and you embrace the safety of a default commitment, bad things will start to manifest. Your eyes will begin to wander because your heart is not fulfilled. Therefore, you are the one who has to speak the truth; don't wait for someone else to be the grown-up. Admit that you have been lying to yourself when you say you're happy when you know you're really not. Tell your co-conspirator that you are going to release them from this fallacy. There is no need to discuss how uninterested you are in pushing your lips against their lips; that's harsh and too specific. Instead, keep it concise: "I need to talk to you about our relationship. I have really enjoyed our time together and I think we were supposed to be in each other's lives, but I need to let you go so that you can find the person who is meant to love you the way you deserve to be loved." That's it.

There is not a lot more to say. If your relationship lacks passion, you need to decide if you're willing to move on in an honest way. Your soul knows what it wants and imprisoning your soul is never a good idea. Again, bad things will happen. The two alternatives to ending a soul-sucking relationship are celibacy (yeah, your spouse is your platonic friend!) or infidelity (yeah, now more lying can happen!).

Being honest isn't easy. Being honest is sometimes very painful. Being honest is the right thing to do. You are meant to have a divinely inspired life while on this planet. You are meant to live with joy, passion, and purpose. Everyone *deserves* romantic love. Everyone deserves to get dizzy-drunk-horny from a kiss. In order to get what you deserve, you have to step up and establish non-negotiable rules for yourself. If you want someone who will inspire your spiritual practice, challenge you intellectually, make you laugh at inappropriate times, and send you cart-wheeling through the cosmos with an orgasm, then set the bar there!

Set your standards today. Say to yourself that you will stay open-minded and receptive to different types of people on dates, but you won't compromise on your expectations. And then actually do it!

Actually break up with someone on the fourth date if the thought of them running their hand down your back makes you queasy. Tell them you don't think you're a good fit for the long haul if their natural smell makes you cringe. Explain that you're not the woman for them if you can't imagine kissing them head to toe. You are setting them free to be with a woman who actually will love their touch, smell and taste. She'll want to cuddle, kiss, and love your ex. Give *her* your ex! Let *her* have your ex!

And then say a prayer that the woman who is currently entangled with the potential love of your life breaks it off in the near future so that your soul can make the connection it was meant to make.

Ladies, we have got to do the right thing so we all can get it on with our super-sexy soul mate.

Step 2: If You're Not Horny-Break-up!!

Let's Get Reflective...

1. **What are the signs you notice in yourself when a romantic relationship is falling flat?**

_____
_____
_____
_____
_____

2. **Why have you stayed in a relationship past its expiration date?**

_____
_____
_____
_____
_____

3. How do you want to feel in an ideal romantic relationship? You can answer this even if you're in a relationship now…it's important to set intentions in order to get results!

_____
_____
_____
_____
_____

4. Describe a couple who seem to have love and lust intermingling.

_____
_____
_____
_____
_____

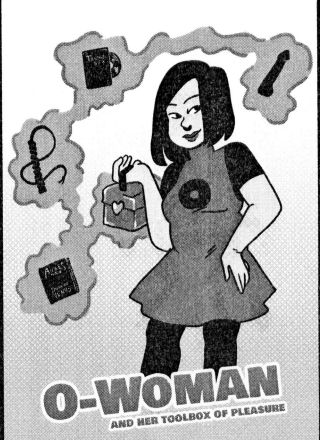

STEP 3

OWN YOUR O

This chapter is dedicated, and written for, my hetero-ladies. According to all of my lesbian friends, this topic is "a straight girl problem" that they found very confusing/amusing.

Let's start off nice and slow with this sensitive subject: Women need to masturbate in order to know their own bodies. Haha, tricked you! This topic is too important to beat around the bush. *pun definitely intended* You have one lifetime in this beautiful body, so don't wait- masturbate!

If you feel like it's dirty or sneaky to do this without your husband/lover, then ask him if he'd mind if you worked on achieving stronger orgasms when he wasn't home so that you could become a better lover. Who would say no to that? He might even surprise you with a vibrator to support your endeavors. Loving partners want a sexual encounter to be magical and that takes *two* explosive reactions, not one. Sex needs balance and one orgasm is just off balance- you need to do your part to even things out!

You have the power, but if you rarely (or never) have an orgasm during intercourse, then you should concede that you're probably not going to figure it out in the midst of the action. You need to do your homework and prepare *in advance*. Special message to those who say "sometimes I climax-if the planets align and he does X, Y, and Z for 25 minutes"…you need to masturbate, too! You need to figure out exactly what your body requires so it's not left to luck.

The point of this whole chapter is to remind you: You are the boss of your own body. No one "gives" you an orgasm. You join an intimate contract with your man when you both agree to engage in a physical expression of your love. At no point should your physical pleasure just randomly pop up like a surprise bouquet of flowers. Instead, it should be as thought out as the emerald cut diamond engagement ring that *you* picked out and had sized to fit your finger perfectly. He can still buy it and place it on your finger, but there was some work involved by both parties.

Your climax or Moment of Euphoric Transcendence (MET) must be initiated and orchestrated by YOU. Your partner is there to facilitate your climactic moment, not to discover it in the back closet of your libido in a dusty box under a bag of clothes ready for Goodwill. Remember: *you* are the boss of *your* body!

Said a different way: Your man knows how to have an orgasm. Every time. He is not dependent on you to figure out what position or scenario will make him achieve his MET. He will move and grab and guide your body until it is in harmony with his. He is the boss of his own body and he knows exactly how to use all the tools in his toolbox; especially his sexual tools. He won't look at you with a dependent, figure-out-how-to-make-me-climax gaze. And aren't you glad? Do you want a lover who knows what he wants and joyfully includes you in the process? Yes! Do you know why he is so attuned to his body? Because he has spent hours and hours masturbating! This started long before you entered his life: the teen years are a busy time of experimentation and ejaculation for males. He learned all the ways he can reach MET and has become confident in his ability to achieve MET *every* time he tries. That confidence is important, too. Just knowing that you can, makes it easier for you to replicate that result.

In The Case of the Female Orgasm (Harvard University Press), researcher Elisabeth Lloyd found that only 25% of women report they consistently have an orgasm during sex. Why?! Ladies, we have no excuse other than our own laziness. With 24 hours in a day, you can spend a mere 20-30 minutes on your orgasm until you can get to MET in less than 5 minutes. Experiment with things that may turn you on: sexy music, water (shower, hot tub jets), standing naked in front of a mirror, porn (print or internet), erotic lit, etc.

I have to laugh when I think about a post like this for men. It would be absurd to talk to men about how they need to learn to achieve an orgasm. They would love a homework assignment that asked them to take time out of each day to masturbate; whereas, many women probably cringed when I suggested it for them. People would assume a male-orgasm chapter was a joke or a clever satire piece.

So why is this message necessary for women? Because of fricking fairy tales, that's why! We all would love to surrender the responsibility of our rescue to a handsome knight in shining armor or his buddy, Prince Charming. Sure we can be sassy and gutsy during the day, but it does feel nice to let someone else take over and take the lead during sex. They can swoop in and resolve the situation; at least that's our hope.

The fact that men like this role *up to a point* is also important to consider. They love the idea of being there for us, giving us what we need that no one else can provide. Let's be real, though, that's a big burden when it comes to the sometimes complex and/or elusive female orgasm. Men want to feel successful and you can help them achieve that goal by doing your part.

Men shouldn't try their hardest and then see your polite "it's fine, honey" smile at the finish line.

The American Psychological Association found that 90% of men want their partner to have an orgasm. They want to go on the adventure with you that ends with your eyes wide open (or shut), screaming or crying, sweating, panting, clawing, slapping, etc and then finally knock-out asleep. If you have MET goals, you should add "passing out in blissful slumber" to the list. You're allowed to fly so high that you crash from exhaustion. No worries about cuddling afterwards- you both know how you feel about each other. Love has been expressed physically, you don't have to belabor the point with additional chitchat or touching.

So. It's time to move beyond the cerebral components of this argument for masturbation and get carnal. Let that sacral chakra know who's boss. You need to figure out what makes you tick so that you can show your man how to wind you up. Learn what pleasure feels like in your own body so you'll be able to recognize and nurture it when your body has become interdependent with another body.

You are meant to be happy and whole during this lifetime. For men and women, sexual expression is normal and natural. You have the tools, you just need to learn how to use them. It's time to experience orgasmic equality. No more shame or frustration or uneven sexual experiences.

Once you have MET with success, you'll realize you've had the power inside you all along. Dorothy would be proud.

Step 3: Own Your O

Let's Get Reflective...

1. What were your impressions of sex as a child? How did that stay the same or evolve through the years?

_____
_____
_____
_____
_____

2. Are you comfortable with the idea/act of masturbation? Why/why not?

_____
_____
_____
_____
_____

3. **List 4 women who seem confident their sexual power:**

_____

_____

_____

_____

4. **If you're in a relationship, go ask your husband/lover what he thinks about you masturbating…I'll wait here…**
Did his answer surprise you?

_____

_____

_____

5. **In what ways would you like to have more "orgasm equality" in your life?**

_____

_____

_____

_____

_____

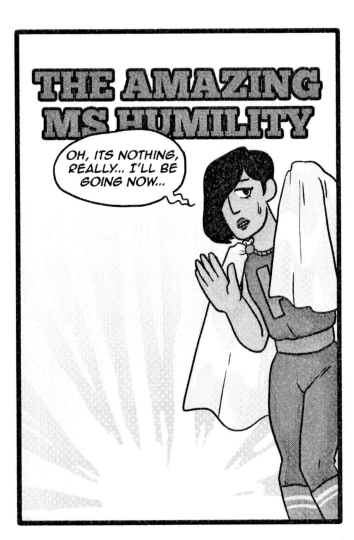

STEP 4

❖

SO LONG, MS. HUMILITY

I am not sorry that I'm going to ask you to be unapologetic. You should be sorry that you say "sorry" so frequently. Women apologize their power away on a regular basis and I'm going to challenge you to become an agent of change. If you can stop apologizing, others stop feeling the need to apologize, too. This mindset shift will change lives and rock your world.

Why? The impact of words is a real factor in people's perceptions of you. We judge others and they judge us, often in very brief interactions. We also evaluate one another based on words alone: emails, memos, text messages, voice messages, and brief conversations. Let's raise our awareness during these speedy interactions and make sure they truly represent us in the best light possible.

We express so much with our choice of language: we share our view of the world by sharing our experiences through an optimistic or pessimistic verbal filter. Furthermore, we tell others about our education and regional background through our subject/verb agreement, emphasis on syllables, and general vocabulary. Finally, we show others how we feel about our self and our role in this lifetime when we apologize for things that aren't really our fault. Some aspects of our speech and language we can control more than others; saying "sorry" habitually is one tendency we all can nip.

I'm bummed that many women apologize because they underestimate their own worthiness. As a society, we tend to place varying levels of worthiness on different jobs. We understand that this is often represented in the form of monetary rewards. The "better" jobs get more lucrative salaries. We show respect for certain positions by changing the titles of those individuals; Mr. or Ms. becomes Dr. and we all recognize the increased worthiness.

While acknowledging the sliding scale of salaries or class rank is not going to change by the time you finish this chapter, you can take inventory of your own worth and adjust your relationship to your role on Earth. If we have the potential to change lives (we all do and will change many lives before we die), then we should admit that we have a pretty intense role to fulfill. Instead of listing all of the worthy, but often overlooked, careers we have in our communities, I'd like to challenge you to look inward and take a breath.

Breath in for 6…hold for 7…exhale for 8.

In that breath you are reaching the depths of your being and feeling the living strength that lies within. That breath is oxygenating your blood and pumping through your veins. That simple inhalation is a meditative prayer that says "You are whole, alive, real, here" and it powers every muscle in your body. That beautiful breath fuels your memories and your future plans. It fills you with another moment of potential in this life. When you want to know your worth, take that breath and feel the unity that you share with every other living creature on this planet. Your worth is inherent and cannot be earned. You cannot lose your worth by making a bad choice. You cannot gain more worth by working late at your job. You do not have the power to change your worth; you were gifted endless potential when you took that first breath and felt the cold reality of life. Worth is inherent. This is not debatable. Now, what to do with all that worth…

Having a strong sense of self-worth means you don't have to be sorry. Our goal is to become so comfortable being yourself that you don't take on other people's energy. You can just be you. It means that you can feel shy, sad, scared, nervous, uncomfortable, or even depressed, but you don't have to be sorry about it. When you get tongue-tied you don't apologize or explain away your lack of verbal fluidity. If you make a mistake at work, accept responsibility without adopting a stance of moral failure. We all make mistakes. You can sleep with a terrible lover (again), wear an unflattering outfit, pick boring movie, or choose a disgusting restaurant without worrying about what anyone else might think. Making mistakes does not jeopardize your self-worth. You can acknowledge that choice wasn't your favorite, but keep it moving. Life isn't about being perfect; it's about making choices and learning from the outcome.

On the other side of gender-land, men will occasionally apologize, but it's not the crutch that "sorry" is for females. Women are also unique in our ability to embrace the indirect apology; we staunchly remain humble even when we should be proud. We shy away from bragging or telling stories that imply we are better, more successful, or more secure than someone else. We do these things for very noble reasons; we don't want to make another woman feel bad about herself. By assuming responsibility for another woman's potential insecurity, we create more uncertainty in ourselves. Instead of opening an opportunity for others to share, celebrate, and prosper *with* us, we live smaller and quieter than necessary. We model that meek is chic.

The most overwhelming challenge comes with collective appreciation. We often dismissively accept praise from others when we are showered with recognition. When it begins to rain love and adoration, we humbly raise a hand and say anyone could have done it.

It was nothing.

I was honored to do the work.

We suck the life out of the compliment with the

shaking of our heads.

It's fine if you're blushing, but don't shut down. Don't clam up!

Stand up straight and smile confidently. Thank everyone for their support. Give a shout-out those who helped you accomplish your goal. Tell everyone how your next project is bigger and better than this one and you're going to need all this positive energy to make it happen. Recycle that enthusiasm and revisit the moment your soul was seen and loved by so many other souls. We can make powerful, soulful connections in these moments if we stay open.

All that being said, apologizing for acts that require genuine contrition are not necessarily included in this step, but can still be analyzed because women tend to adopt more responsibility than necessary when they do something "wrong." Rudeness falls into this ambiguous category; 90% of us (totally made-up statistic) feel rude when we hurt someone's feelings.

Case in point: we want to speak our mind, but then are overcome with guilt for making someone else feel uncomfortable feelings (anger, defensiveness, shame). This is a tough area for us to critique, but I'm here to tell you that you are not responsible for other women's feelings. My mantra has always been to speak my truth with love and kindness and then allow the receiver to process the information with the tools at their disposal. When we add a layer of apologies on top of a blunt cup of real-talk, it is not only confusing, but the "I'm so sorry, but…" often contradicts the message you're trying to convey.

Example: You may need tell me that it would be better for our business if other members of the steering committee have a chance to share more of their insight. (Oops, I must be dominating a lot of committee meeting discussions!) At first I'm feeling embarrassed… and that's fine! I should be a little embarrassed that I didn't notice others weren't getting a chance to speak. The hope is that I'm secure enough in myself that I can eventually smile and reply, "message received!" to the person brave enough to advocate for the group.

How amazing would it be to then thank the person giving the feedback and emulate their ability to speak their mind in my own life. On the flip side, if

I had apologized profusely and started to tailspin into a shame vortex, the speaker may feel compelled to wrap me in a blanket of insincere apologizes for upsetting me. It would be an, "I'm sorry." "No, I'm sorry" game of tag!

Ideally, both parties should strive to speak with loving candor and process the situation through their own filters. Don't operate from a place of uncertainty and don't make someone else's insecurity your responsibility. Live with holy, loving intentions and everything will come out exactly as it should. Again, folks might get upset when you speak your truth, but that is not your fault.

*Note: If someone gives you feedback that you do *not* find enlightening, there may be room to ask clarifying questions or to flatly reject the speaker's perspective. This is where your gut will kick in and let you know what the truth actual is in this particular case. When you allow your ego to take a nap, your consciousness or soul will show up with wisdom and guidance.

I hope you see that saying you're sorry throughout your day and in every circumstance that is uncomfortable, is not representing your worth. It may seem small, but this is a huge block for many of us. You are a model woman. You must stand strong, proud, and confident in your worth. The words "I'm sorry" convey a stance that is diminished, weak, and lacking. "I am sorry" sounds like I'm flawed/imperfect/damaged on a subconscious level and does not allow your essence to radiate.

So back to real life: you look a mess. Okay! Don't say you're sorry you look bad. Maybe your house or car or career or boyfriend or landscaping is un-kept; don't apologize your way through it. Laugh and acknowledge your situation and keep the worth that you inherently have.

Moms, don't apologize for your kids when they are being their normal, happy (rambunctious) selves. My favorite mom-friends smile and revel in their children's natural expressions of joy. Their detachment from the desire for a child's submissive obedience frees me as a mom. I am then more likely to embrace the exuberance of my three young sons. Furthermore, give children the appropriate venues to be awesome and cheer them on! They need to know their worth, too! Often, removing pressure on yourself and your kids to be perfect makes everyone feel better.

From work, to home, to relationships, let's all agree to say, "So long, Sorry Sally!" We are here to shine our light for the whole world to see. Our radiant presence is the gift we give to other women. We lead by example and invite all of our sisters to live with loving intentions and speak the truth that demonstrates our individual and collective worth.

Step 4: So Long, Ms. Humility

Let's Get Reflective...

1. Describe a situation (or two) when you've heard a woman say "I'm sorry" when it wasn't needed.

   _____
   _____
   _____
   _____
   _____

2. Do you say "I'm sorry" when you could say "excuse me"?   YES   NO

3. When do you observe men saying "I'm sorry"?

   _____
   _____
   _____
   _____
   _____

4. Describe a time when you could have received recognition more graciously. If you dismissively accepted praise, how would you re-do the situation if you could go back?

_____
_____
_____
_____
_____

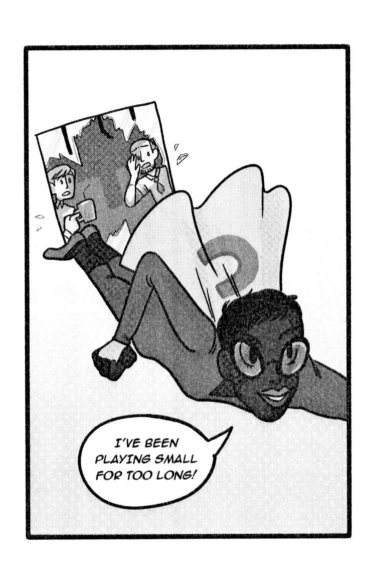

STEP 5

❖

BLOW SOME SHIT UP!

It's time to do some demo work; time to blow up some stuff. We are going to mess around with aspects of your life that you don't think about very often. Let's start off with a little negativity to get you headed in the right direction; let's assume you're nowhere near your potential. You have a life that provides you with the level of comfort that you feel you deserve, but you are living within your snuggly, safe zone. Let's extend the premise even farther; I bet you don't even think about your potential because you are too busy living life. Don't worry, it's not totally your fault.

No one asks you anymore what you want to be when you grow up. There are no whimsical conversations about being President or an astronaut; you are what you are. You are you right now and there are no fanciful plans for the future. That's not to say you don't have highlights on the horizon: fun vacations, big birthday celebrations, weddings, births, moving into nicer houses.

That is all really important stuff. It is. But what if you put the "normal" life stuff on the backburner for a moment and daydreamed. If you love your job, try to fantasize about a version of your job that would be even more amazing. Would you travel (all expenses paid)? Maybe work from home some days or just work less hours? Could you stand to have more/less responsibilities? Would you like your job a smidge more if your salary increased, you had more vacation time, or better benefits? How about a work environment that encouraged personal growth, attention to wellness, or creative outlets?

You say you actually dread your job!? For you folks, we're going to play a game where you get "fantasy fired" from your current place of employment. Now that you're pretend-unemployed, you have to design the perfect job that will marry your skills and passion with a real need in society. Imagine your ideal salary because that's what you're going to make in this made-up world. What do you do in your perfect job? Where do you go each day and how do you feel in this new role?

We're focusing on jobs for this reflection because jobs are an easy place to start pushing our potential. We can objectively assess our level of engagement and enjoyment because we spend a lot of time at work. That being said, there are several factors that may skew your assessment of your current (real) employment. If you make a decent salary, have a convenient commute, and love your job security, it will be hard to seriously consider other options.

Back to our game: Let's remove salary from the equation because we are pretending we make the perfect salary already. A convenient commute is great if your life expectations align with minimal effort. A quick commute or working from home only counts as a perk if you like to start your workday quick and easy. If you don't dig your current career, I wouldn't count getting there quickly as a benefit. Job security is tricky because it is like a full-bodied hug; sweet and comforting, unless you don't really like the person who is hugging you.

Why celebrate your ability to stay in a job that you don't like in the first place? Furthermore, the last factor is bred in fear of the current job market. We often compare what we have to what others don't have and then pile heaps of gratitude onto our situation. "Lord, I'm so glad I have a job that is mildly inspiring because there are so many unemployed people in the world. Amen." This gives us a false sense of accomplishment because we have what others don't have. The job market in any country will always be challenging, but I want to challenge you to start a shift in your thinking away from scarcity. We are meant to live bigger. You are meant to live in abundance. Consider what you *can* have as opposed to what others *don't* have.

You were on the right track as a kid when you dreamed of flying to outer space or penning a best-selling novel. You were aiming for awesome when you cast yourself in an imaginary movie or surgically replaced your little brother's heart with kitchen tongs during a play-surgery. Did you race around the house and win a gold medal in the Olympics? Design an eco-friendly home using paper out of the computer printer and a #2 pencil?

When you pretended to be amazing, you felt amazing. Your field of potential was huge and your energy was charged. You were living as if you were already in these roles and on some level, your soul smiled.

Your responsibility is to live life at a high vibration. You achieve this level of energy when you are engaged in work that is aligned with your soul. If you think about your current job and you notice that you are not buzzing with excitement, then you may need to start fantasizing again. Daydream in your mind, your journal/diary, in fiction writing, on a vision board, over coffee with your best friend, or with children.

Side note: children are extremely supportive of dreamers. They will ask important follow-up questions about your dream job like: "Could you ride on a zebra during your business trip?" "How will you help people?" "What could you invent?" "Will you make a million billion dollars?" "Could you be on TV?" They love to pretend and they love to laugh. Living at a higher vibration demands creative energy and joyful presence; kids are great teachers in this area.

So, back to our game…

What's next?

After you dream out loud in some fashion, you are going to be faced with the very real possibility that you have expectations of greatness for yourself. You may realize that you have some very real potential, young lady! When you allow yourself to think about how you can blend pleasure, purpose, and passion, you might end up with a goal that is a little (or A LOT) scary to you right now. The key is not to smother your dreams with the pillow of self-doubt.

Our ego loves to undermine our genius and hand us a weapon to quiet our inner-voice of awesomeness. You may actually hear yourself say: "That was so stupid to think I could do that." "Who am I to think I could actually do something that risky?" "Why did I waste my time daydreaming about something that will never come true? Now I just feel bad."

It's so important that we understand that the mean thoughts we have about ourselves isn't really us. We need to acknowledge those thoughts for what they are: the ego, fear, and insecurity. We can quiet them with the same love we would use to soothe a child or comfort a friend. We can gently extend a hand to our nervous inner-child and take a step forward. Just take one step; no leaping necessary. After that you will intuitively know how to move in the direction of your dreams. Some part of your personal genius will tell you what you need to do to learn more about your ideal life. In some area of your heart you will hear a whisper and you'll know who your cheerleaders will be; look to them for help. Eventually, aspects of your life will open up so wide that opportunities will begin to appear every time you take a step in the right direction.

You have been good for so long in this lifetime. You have worked so hard. It's time to blow some sh#*t up and break out of the groove that has gotten predictable. Get out there and live a little bigger. When you are aligned with your high-vibration calling, you will get the promotion, find the new job, step into a leadership role, go on an unscripted adventure, or have passionate love in your life.

Peek around the corner of your life and see where you're headed. Then take one step in that direction.

Just one step.

Then another.

Step 5: Blow Some Shit Up!

Let's Get Reflective...

1. **What were your dream jobs as a kid:**
    - _____
    - _____
    - _____
    - _____

2. **Describe your perfect job:**

    _____
    _____
    _____
    _____
    _____

3. **Where do you go each day?**

    _____
    _____
    _____
    _____
    _____

4. **How do you feel in this new role?**

   _____
   _____
   _____
   _____
   _____

5. **List your ideal salary for your perfect job:**

   _____

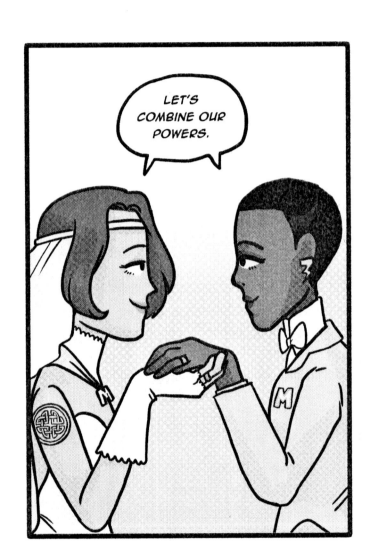

STEP 6

❖

GET MARRIED...OR NOT

"A long marriage is two people trying to dance a duet and two solos at the same time."
–Anne Taylor Fleming

"Love may be blind, but marriage is a real eye-opener."
–Unknown

Women are often conflicted about the *need* to get married. Society has backed away from using the term "spinster," but marriage is still considered a desirable status for women once they reach their mid-twenties. There is not as much pressure for men to commit to marriage at this age, possibly because their ability to reproduce and create a family has a much bigger window than that of a woman. Regardless, the idea that a woman "should" get married has built-in burdens of its own.

Here's a quick exercise we can do to get some clarity on this issue: write 2-3 sentences about the purpose of marriage. In general, why do people get married? (You have space to write your answers at the end of the chapter.) Obviously this answer will reflect your personal philosophy about marriage. If you feel like marriage is a way for two insecure people to confirm their existence on this planet, holy matrimony might not be a worthy pursuit for you at this time. If you think, like me, that marriage is partnership between two people who want to support each other as they go through personal growth, then maybe you're ready to start attracting a mate. There are many, many other philosophies surrounding marriage based on religion, culture, and personal experiences. That being said, the idea of uniting with someone in a formal way is universally acknowledged as a big deal. No one flippantly says we should get married for the weekend or suggests marriage is an easy endeavor. As a society, we respect the idea of marriage as being a major decision.

So is it the right decision for every woman? Short answer: no. Not all women want to be married and many of those women resent the idea that they are counterculture for feeling this way. As a collective, we women are increasing our expectations for relationships and refusing to settle. Married life is one of constant compromise, but not selling-out. More and more females realize that they want personal freedom first and marriage only if that freedom can be preserved. We want our individuality to be celebrated, not endured. This takes a very special spouse and attracting that person requires a higher level of consciousness.

There is no way around it; attracting a spouse is a spiritual practice. It is an ongoing process of opening up your soul and aligning with a partner who is equally interested in traveling through the human life cycle with you. It's critical to understand that human perfection or saving someone are not appropriate expectations going into a marriage.

Instead, we need to commit to the relationship as whole individuals who have strengths and weaknesses that will contribute to the growth of both lives. The vulnerability required in a committed relationship is where the spirituality comes in; allowing someone to see *all of you* is an act of faith. You need faith to reassure your cynical mind that when things get ugly, the other person will not just run out of your life.

In fact, the commitment to simply stay during the times when it would be easier to leave is the biggest part of marriage. There are definitely going to be icky, awkward times: when you realize you don't want to finish the college degree you've paid for, you are having a miscarriage (again), you don't like all of his relatives, you hate her long hours at work, or you feel like you need to change your career. The infrastructure of your marriage should be strong enough to stand in spite of all of the uncertainties. The act of staying is even more important than the talking. Literally staying in the room is the most powerful way to show you want a partner in this journey. You both stay…and then, at some point, you talk. Your commitment to be in the room allows the trust to remain intact and the conversation, even the yelling and crying, to happen.

Attracting the right spouse is key because that person is meant to inspire your growth and growth can come in a lot of different forms. If you find yourself attracting people who push you to learn and grow through conflict and antagonism, you should question whether you want that energy in your life for decades to come. On the flip side, a spouse who triggers you, but is also willing to lovingly address the issues that you need to heal, is a beautiful gift. We should all pray to attract many people in our lives who push us forward while also walking by our side.

For many of us, friends and family members may be all the support we need to grow. The commitment we make to those we have chosen to surround ourselves with is just as important as marriage. If marriage does not resonate with you, sister-friends, siblings or parents may be the fulfilling relationships you need to foster growth. Your independent life with lovers, family, and friends around you could be your ideal path. The next step is to find peace with your choice. As women, we need to honor the choices others make and we need to respect our own choices as well. If you choose not to marry, model confidence for other women who may also be considering the same experience. Embrace the joy that comes with living your true calling and resist adopting any of the fear others may project onto you.

This one lifetime affords us so many opportunities to experience love and support. Stay aligned with the positive energy around you focus on what you want to create. Find peace and satisfaction in the abundance right in front of you each day: so many people you can connect to, learn from, and grow with every single day.

Marriage is just one way to enjoy the human connection and many people find fulfillment in other relationships outside of marriage. Choose your path one step at a time and live in your truth with enthusiasm.

Step 6: Get Married...or Not

Let's Get Reflective...

1. What is the purpose of marriage?

   _____
   _____
   _____
   _____
   _____

2. Why do people get married?

   _____
   _____
   _____
   _____
   _____

3. What relationships or partnerships already exist in your life?
   - ❖ _____
   - ❖ _____
   - ❖ _____

❖ _____
❖ _____

4. Did you always imagine you would get married? Why or why not?

_____
_____
_____
_____
_____

5. If you want to get married, what steps are you taking to allow that relationship to develop in your life?

_____
_____
_____
_____
_____

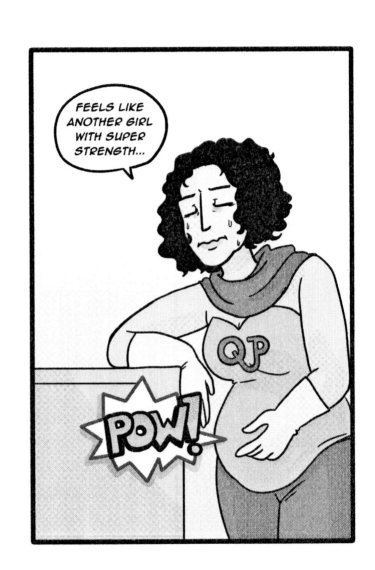

STEP 7

❖

HAVE KIDS...OR NOT

Your children are not your children, they come through you, but they are life itself, wanting to express itself.
– Wayne Dyer

"Having a child is like getting a tattoo...on your face. You better be committed."
–Eat, Pray Love screenplay

Children are wonderful gifts. They bring laughter, gratitude, and awareness to every single day of our life with them. Children teach us how they see the world and how to be more present in our world. They give us a chance to share our life experiences with them and we both grow from the opportunity to do so. Kids are great.

Children are huge responsibilities. They demand our time, energy, and resources every single day. Children will try our patience and challenge our sense of balance. They want love, attention, and guidance even when we don't have those things for our self or our spouse. Kids are frustrating.

There are so many contributing pros and cons to parenthood that the assumption that everyone will reproduce and create a family is baffling. There is no doubt that as a society we have a default assumption that everyone will have, or try to have, a family by the age of 35. Those expectations obviously highest for married couples. It has become a part of our life cycle, despite how evolved we are as a species, to assume everyone has the same inherent, biological desires.

As we are evolving as a species and a culture, expectations are changing. Many folks are marrying later and couples are making the choice to remain childless. This is an important choice that is worth analyzing from a female perspective. All young girls receive messages that romance, marriage, maintaining a house, and becoming a mother are positive aspects of adulthood. It is discussed within the family, shown in the toys available in stores, and played out in movies across the world. We generally frame the discussion as an opt-out scenario; folks choose *not* to get married or *not* to have kids. This is unfortunate; a more heart-centered conversation starts when we ask if we're called to be married or to be parents in the first place.

Considering parenting a spiritual calling is radical. Entering the priesthood, becoming a nun, choosing to become a church minister are all obviously spiritual callings. We acknowledge these commitments come after a long discernment process that involves prayer and self-reflection. Leaders in the field are often called upon to work with a potential candidate to see if he or she is truly meant for the vocation. The process is thoughtful and exhaustive.

Conversely, people become parents through a variety of situational circumstances. Putting aside accidental pregnancy, many parents enter the commitment of raising a child with full consent. The baby is welcomed and parenthood is considered a blessing. This is wonderful! Parenthood is a conscious-raising undertaking and should be made with clear-headed awareness. Furthermore, the decision should only be made by the specific people who are going to be with the child on a daily basis. In other words, communities should be careful not to pressure couples to reproduce if that's not their calling. Societal expectations around the world have normalized comments like, "Why don't you guys have a baby?" "You better hurry up and have kids!" "Who is going to take care of you when you get old?" and this, obviously, puts additional pressure on couples who were not comfortable with the idea of having children. Childless couples are considered abnormal in many circles; couples in most situations have children. While it may be the norm, it does not mean it has to be your normal!

Once you have a baby, you are a parent for life. Pregnancy or adoption is just the opening credits to a very, very long movie. You will spend many hours a day with your child for the rest of your life. You will be challenged to grow in patience, creativity, understanding, and resourcefulness in a way no adult will ever demand of you. There are many gifts and lessons along the way, but they are not available to all parents. You are only eligible for these gifts and lessons if you are awake enough to receive them.

Choosing to be a conscious parent is the most important choice of all. Regardless of how you ended up a parent, we can choose whether we will be present with our children. Will we look them in the eyes? Do we understand their fears or confusion? Can we make the time to show them how to do something before we expect perfection? Do we light up with love when we see our child? Will we focus on their strengths and gifts? Can we trust them to make the right choices? These are daily tasks we must face if we want to stay connected with our children on a soul level. Beyond keeping them alive with food and shelter, parents should be soulfully present as much as possible. Laughing at their jokes that have jumbled punch lines, reading favorite books until the binding dissolves, playing the mind-numbing games they enjoy, and preparing messy meals together are all simple ways to be a conscious parent. Allowing TV or electronic devices to dominate our days is the easiest way to become disconnected with our little ones. The good news? We can decide each and every day how we are going to show up as parents in our children's lives. Yesterday was important, but today is more important. Make sure you get today right.

There isn't a lot more to say about the choice of parenthood other than to emphasize that it is a choice. Don't allow anyone else's expectations determine your future. If they want to be parents, God bless. Hopefully they made a thoughtful commitment to raising children and are actively engaged in family life. That being said, there is no guilt or shame in making a different choice for your life. You are stuck with you for the rest of your days. You must be very reflective about who you allow to stick with you on this journey. Pray, meditate, write, research, babysit, discuss and observe others until you come to a decision that gives you a sense of peace in your heart. Then stand by your choice with loving firmness.

We are meant to live big, messy, fun, sad, silly, scary, happy lives. Every life has a different path and different companions along the way. You have my permission (which may not hold up in a court of law) to confidently declare your path and determine your companions on your own terms. It is your right to be happy, with or without children of your own.

Step 7: Have Kids...or Not

Let's Get Reflective...

1. **Who pressures you regarding off-spring?**

_____

_____

_____

_____

_____

2. **Do you want to have children? Why or why not?**

_____

_____

_____

_____

_____

3. How do you stay engaged when you're interacting with youngsters?

_____

_____

_____

_____

_____

4. What supports do you have as parent?

_____

_____

_____

_____

_____

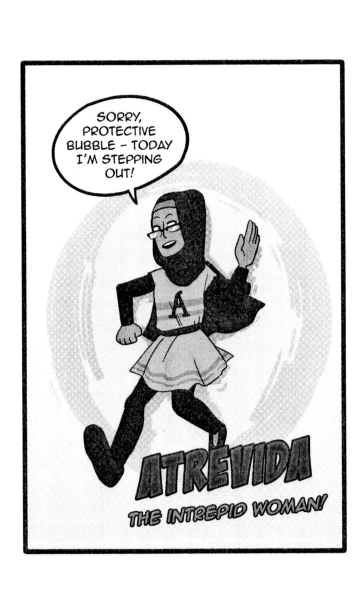

STEP 8

❖

MAKE YOUR ESCAPE PLAN

It's time to take steps in a new direction. You are not going to abandon everything you love, but you are going to set out on a different path. Just for today. You are going to go by yourself to a new coffee shop and you are going to chose a beverage that you have never tasted before. You will drink it and read a magazine, or stare off into space, or watch Mother Nature out the window, or gaze at your coffee while you listen in on the conversation happening at the next table over. You are going to escape your normal routine for about 30 minutes. It's okay if you don't like coffee. Coffee shops have lots of beverages and I'm sure you drink beverages of some type. The point of this is not to hydrate or spy on others, it's to simply take a step in a different direction. That being said, if you always go to coffee shops then you're going to need to make a plan that stretches you a bit. First Aid/CPR training? A book club with strangers at the library? Eating at a restaurant alone? A free intro yoga/pilates/kickboxing/meditation class?

It's less about what you specifically do and more about doing ONE THING that makes you feel a little uncomfortable. If you're excited and super relaxed about your outing, it may be too safe. Stretching exercises like these are meant to push you more than you usually want to go. Instead of brainstorming what you want to do, scan local papers or flyers and try something you never even knew existed. Make your escape plan and stick to it.

You should experience some mild anxiety, or at least, uneasiness before your leave. Questioning whether it is a good idea, how you'll find your location, what you'll do if you're miserable or unhappy is a sign that you're on the right path. Listen politely to your inner voice (hello, ego!) for a moment or two and then move on with life. You don't need to take advice from your inner insecurities; instead push past your fears and just do it anyway.

Go! Go! Go!

Stay present the entire time you are out and about; avoid using your phone or even looking at your phone. Maybe just leave it at home, actually. When you are in a new environment the first thing you'll notice is the energy. Decide what you like or don't like about the vibe you're picking up. Décor and physical surroundings are contributors, but often the humans present impact the energy greatly. Notice how you feel physically in the space. Are you cozy and snug? Surprisingly comfortable after all of your apprehension? Maybe you're somewhat exposed in the middle of a large room or space where you don't know anyone or the routines of the group. How long does it take for you to understand the norms? How long does it take you to feel like you fit in?

As a society, we encourage our children to try new things, go places they've never been before, and interact with people in situations where they do not know the norms. We know it's good for them and we also know that they may initially feel shy or uncertain about what they're supposed to do. But we push them anyway. They survive, and ultimately thrive, by being exposed to new and different experiences.

The lesson children ultimately learn is the one that *you* need to remember: the purpose of life is to try new things, explore your world, and learn as much as you can about the human existence. While it's not mandatory to try new things on a regular basis, if you do, you will learn amazing lessons everyday. You'll see different kinds of love, notice beauty in unexpected places, and hear emotions that you may never have felt yourself. You'll also get the reassuring gift of survival. When you survive your solo adventure, you teach your mind that the ego doesn't always know what's best for you. Ultimately you realize that being uncomfortable doesn't mean you shouldn't do something.

Quick side-note: I am a firm believer in intuition and "trusting your gut," pay attention to any alerts you receive, everyday, everywhere. Gauge whether you need to alter plans or avoid certain people. Hypothetical fears feel different than actual bone-chilling signs from your internal compass. Listen to your compass when you're in a space that feels threatening or unsafe.

Our human lifetime is a momentary circumstance that you are meant to enjoy. Getting out of your routine is one of the fastest ways to jumpstart high-energy alignment. Connecting with universal energy is an easy way to stay engaged and happy with each day of your life. Being in new places with new people will allow you to grow and expand faster than staying in your lane and playing small.

Today is the day. Stretch, grow, expand, learn, love, laugh! Then you die. Life is awesome. Get out there and see what you've been missing!

Step 8: Make Your Escape Plan

Let's Get Reflective...

1. What's the last routine-busting thing you've done?

   _____
   _____
   _____
   _____
   _____

2. Think of 3 places you could go to make you nervous/excited and a little uncomfortable:

   o _____
   o _____
   o _____

3. Go to at least one place listed above...I'll wait...

4. How was your adventure?

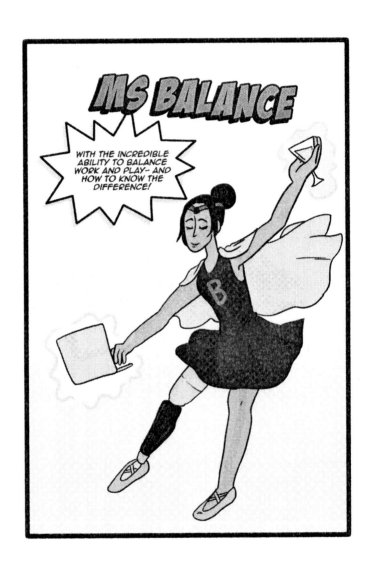

STEP 9

❖

YOUR STRESS AIN'T CUTE

"Hey, how are you?!"

"Oh, good; busy though."

And thus begins a conversation around a list of things that have to be done, usually all before the sun sets that evening. Work, kids, shopping, more kids, prep for tomorrow's day at work… I get it; you're a very busy person. You are so busy that when I ask about yourself, you proactively define yourself by your to-do list. I used to be mildly offended when people; mostly women, subjected me to their detailed run-down of activities. It seemed designed to inform me how they were busy and important while I was not. I assumed that their responses implied they were busy because they were good workers, mothers, friends, volunteers, etc. while I was slacking off and making more work for women like them.

No fear, I have since gotten over myself. It's highly unlikely that frazzled women who wanted to vent to a nice person who asked about their day were actually trying to make me feel inferior. Furthermore, I know that I'm busy, too. I also know that simply being busy doesn't make me a good mom, friend, worker, or volunteer. Most of the time it just means I over-committed to things that sounded like a good idea when it was proposed to me. We want to live a fun, bigger life, but it's hard to gauge when saying yes to promising opportunities will demand that we repeatedly have to say no to ourselves along the way.

There are a lot of messages in the fem-sphere that tell women to learn how to say "no" to people. It's an important skill, but I worry that saying "no" is a short-sighted. You want to be open to opportunities, but they have to feel good. Feeling is a key signal that our bodies give us to steer us to our dharma or path. We need to align ourselves with the emotions and feelings that present themselves to us. Do we feel like this will be a fun experience that will stretch us and help us grow? Are we only doing this because it is the right thing to do and someone should do it? One is a high energy question and the other is most definitely a low energy question.

Here's the solution: everyone should do what makes her heart come alive. If we could all commit to that, then every job would be filled and every committee would be packed (or the role would vanish due to lack of interest). There is a time and place for you to volunteer at an event that you would enjoy as much as the participants. I love reading and writing, maybe you love jogging and tennis. Let's not try to do each other's passion projects. I don't want to be the leader of a jogging or tennis club. You may not want to lead teen book clubs or writing workshops (I love doing both of these things!) and that's okay. If we all experiment with our interests and find a good fit, everyone will benefit from human interactions that aren't sprinkled with complaints about busyness, but instead, have a passionate leadership.

"But the children!" Ahh, the children must be driven here and there and given opportunities to swim, and play soccer, and draw, and practice their instruments, and have play dates, and go camping! We must teach them how to manage their packed calendars so they can learn to be as busy as we are as adults. They must learn how days start early, run at a ragged pace, and end late with rushed meals throughout. It's for their own good that they get to experience so many wonderful clubs and organizations. It is important for their college application; being well-rounded is an asset. Maybe.

The idea of slowing down childhood has been discussed in various venues with the main argument resting on the concept of unstructured time. The free time kids get when they're not in school is ideal for rest, play, reading, drawing, writing, play, daydreams, exploring, play, tag, play, play, play.

Study after study show that children thrive in school when they are able to play and explore before the age of 5. Youth is meant to be carefree, but I would argue that adulthood has that potential too. This is a trickier case to make because of the added responsibilities of work, home, and family. My only point in this debate around hyper-busyness is that we all have the power to set priorities. If your priorities demand that you work long hours in order to make a lot of money to pay for the things that you want, then you will not be relaxing very often.

If you choose to focus on your job, spouse, children or friends, more than yourself, then you will not prioritize self-care. If you feel most worthy when you give every part of yourself away to your church, family, friends, or a job, then you won't be willing to schedule time alone doing things you love when you even do have the time to do them. You won't want to meditate, bathe, get a massage, read a book, enjoy a movie, savor a meal in silence or play around in your garden because it will feel like your wasting time. When we prioritize other things over ourselves we no longer "feel" good when we try to take time to do things we love. Some of us even feel guilty that we are "just sitting around"…what?! Why is sitting so extravagant that we can't give ourselves time each day to just enjoy our leisure?

Maybe I wouldn't be so sure that self-care is lacking in contemporary society if my busy friends seemed happy. They are lovely women who smile a lot, but I work with too many female clients not to know the truth. Most feel that they are tired and worn out by the existence they have created for themselves. Stress is such a common complaint that most women dismiss because they know many other women feel the same way; it's become normalized.

Let's sit with the concept of stress for another moment. Stress is not normal when it's constant. You should not be in a constant state of stress. Women who have experienced life-threatening circumstances related to violence or extreme deprivation must also endure the constant stress of trying to survive, but that should never become the norm for most women on the planet. The number of American women who do not get a healthy night's rest is distressing. We are staying up late and getting up early with pockets of insomnia wreaking havoc on our REM sleep. The deep, restorative sleep that we need to maintain health and sanity is sabotaged by worry, anticipation, insecurities, and fears. We can't sleep because we are trying to manage more things than necessary.

The first step to restoring balance is to revisit priorities; what do we want out of life? Family time, a big house, a new car, the kids in a fancy school, a promotion at work? What is the goal we are working to achieve?

If you know that you cannot sustain your level of stress you are currently under for the next year, then you should not try to endure it for even the next week. Stress has a direct impact on your physical existence; when you hear folks talking about manifesting illness, injury, and disease, it's not mystical mumbo-jumbo. Your tense muscles lead to cramping, spasms, bone misalignment, headaches, and more. Your anxiety has an impact on your food choices and healthy digestion. Because your overall health is regulated through your gut, many diseases begin with digestion and nutrient absorption. Illness is inevitable when high levels of stress are present. Even lack of sleep will deplete the body of its ability to maintain basic levels of health; stressed out people are bound to get sick.

The question isn't when you will get sick, but how bad your wake-up call will need to be before you pick up the phone and have a conversation with yourself about changing your priorities. A cold or even the flu may be easy to dismiss, a migraine or extra weight gain might be concerning, but some of us will sustain an injury or discover a disease before we reflect on our stress levels.

Don't allow yourself to be a victim of your own priorities! Consciously decide what you want and need in life. Set goals that you can work towards over time. Stay in-tune with the rhythms of your body and give yourself a DNA boost: Decent sleep, Nutritious food, and an Active lifestyle. Nuture relationships and savor the present moment. If you have a busy life because of your ambitious priorities, own it! Allow the abundance of your days to energize you and fill you with gratitude. I'm often very busy, but I love it! I think it's cool to hang out with so many different people and experience so many varied activities. When I get overwhelmed I step back and veg out. I'm no party animal, so most of my nights are quiet from 8pm on. I stay up late sometimes, but I'm usually reading, writing, watching TV, or making out with my husband. I'm definitely not working, stressing, or cleaning. Ick!

Your stress ain't cute, but you are! You are so flipping adorable that people love being around you. You are in demand *because* of your gifts and personality. You, strong lady, are a powerful ruler; you are a Queen. You are the only Queen of your kingdom, which is pretty amazing. It's important to decide each day how you're going to rule your vast kingdom. Make the choices that bring you joy and light you up. Be the Queen who inspires others to rule with power and grace as well.

Step 9: Your Stress Ain't Cute

Let's Get Reflective...

1. Describe how stress shows up in your life:

   _____
   _____
   _____
   _____
   _____

2. List 5 things you wish you didn't "have to do":

   ➢ _____
   ➢ _____
   ➢ _____
   ➢ _____
   ➢ _____

3. Think about your power to prioritize. What activities can you let go of that don't "light you up" when you include them in your day? *Remember: it's a big kingdom, but you're the Queen.*

_____
_____
_____
_____
_____

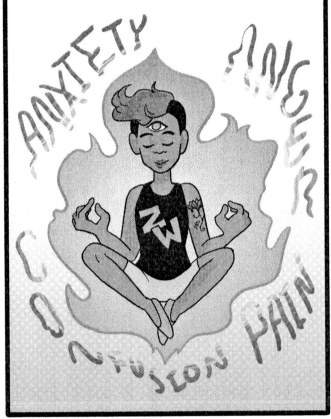

STEP 10

❖

MEDITATE OR DIE

So we acknowledge that noise and busyness often fill our days. We thrive on the activities we schedule for ourselves and we dedicate our lives looking for happiness, peace, and purpose. The daily onslaught of stress-inducing work, errands, relationships, and home life never stops. Aside from sleep, our days are filled with the buzz of actions and reactions. We live, learn, respond, and make decisions in an endless cycle.

Your spirit is extremely taxed in the midst of high-stress living. It wants to be calm and peaceful, but is either on high-alert or ignored by your egoic mind that demands more and more. In our effort to find peace we look for remedies that can come in two, dangerous (yet popular) forms: medication and alcohol. While both of these can soothe us in the short term, extended addictions are not the foundation of inner peace. We cannot rely on external resources to heal our internal pain; the response must be aligned with the cause.

Our disconnection with our spiritual selves is often the root cause of suffering. We know we're not happy, but we're not sure why. We look at our spouse, children, house, car, job, friends, and even our own physical body. We ask why aren't these things good enough? Why aren't they better? We want our spouse to be more attentive. Our children should be more obedient. Our house and car are not exactly the style we want or they aren't as clean or new as they could be. Our job? Colleagues are lazy, our boss is a nag and the commute is ruining our lives. Friends are great, but so demanding yet rarely available when we need them. Let's not even start on our body! Our body is so disappointing. We lack the tone, definition, physique, shape, color, or size that we deserve. If only we had the perfect body then we wouldn't feel so discontent with life.

That is a long list of complaints, ladies. Change for many of us could easily include a lot of factors outside of ourselves; many external components that have nothing to do with your soul, spirit, mind, or heart. It is both frustrating and a relief to have these "shortcomings" fall on the laps of our spouse or our boss. It's not our fault that our kids are bad and the neighborhood is unsatisfactory. In our mind, we have been stuck with some terrible circumstances. The idea that we are surviving it all is commendable, actually!

What if the response to pain and frustration relied less on material factors and medication and was instead linked to something you could actually influence? What if you had the power to change your circumstances without any action from the people or aspects of your life that cause you stress? What if you could rid yourself of unhappiness all by yourself?

If you read the title of this chapter, you can probably predict that I'm going to recommend meditation to solve all of your problems. It's true. Meditation is the first step in the direction of rebooting your life. When you feel anxious, angry, insecure, or even lonely, meditation will help you transcend the negative moment.

Somehow sitting in silence allows a certain level of peace to enter your life. When you carve out time to focus on yourself and your peace you send a message to your subconscious that you are worthy of care. Through meditation you elevate your worthiness in your own mind. Self-care has so many benefits, but one of the overlooked perks is that you are communicating with yourself that you actually matter. You deserve time just like all of the other people in your life. You can forge a way forward through trying times when you respect your own need for nourishment; when you take time to heal emotionally.

While soulful healing is not guaranteed during any particular moment of silence, meditation adds a layer of focus that facilitates the potential for loving rejuvenation. When you meditate, you start in a state of openness; you demonstrate a desire to allow peace in your day. You then find a way to be comfortable, usually sitting, and open your palms upward to physically mirror your mental state of allowing.

Breathing is often taken for granted and ignored in our daily lives, but during meditation you are going to be aware of your inhales… and…your exhales. Some people prefer to *only* focus on their breath during meditation, while others take note of their breathing and then move on to a mantra or meaningful saying that they repeat silently. Regardless, taking time to feel and appreciate your life-giving breath automatically makes you more aware of your being. The natural tendency is to take a deep inhalation and then a slow exhalation when you're actually tuned into your breath. Your body instantly feels a boost from the conscious breathing and you may want to repeat it a few more times.

This quick, intuitive, exercise often leads to a desire to stretch. You may open your eyes, yawn, spread your arms, flex your toes, or twist your trunk. More oxygen in your body inspires other natural reflexes that lead to physical alignment. Breathing during meditation helps you stay focused on clearing your mind, repeating a mantra, or absorbing the message of a guided meditation. This one component of meditation will remind you how easy it is to get connected to our bodies and simply feel better without much effort.

Beyond comfort and breathing, meditation

requires that you focus on something other than ego. Your ego is the voice in your head that tells you what to do, what to think about things, and how you should live your life. Your ego keeps you engaged in the human experience, but it needs to take a break sometimes. Once you can quiet your mind (your ego), you will be able to recharge yourself in a way you may never have experienced before. This isn't the same as sleeping; we stay awake and aware during meditation. Our focus is on something beyond the chatter in our brain, however. We start in a place of comfort where we are physical open, then we get attuned to our body through breathing, and finally, we devote our entire focus to the quiet *beyond* our thoughts.

Meditation truly happens when we slow everything down and feel our soul's connection to all things. We remember the genesis of our being and we have a release from our material world. In a meditative state you understand that your car, house, family, job, and body exist, but they don't define you. You understand that you have attracted all of these things into your human experience through your energy and your choices. You comprehend that there are lessons to be learned from your unique time on Earth. But you are not Earthbound. There is so much more than being an Earthling. You are so much more that your body, your job, your successes, and your failures. You are energy - light - love.

It is difficult to write about the experience of meditation, that's why it needs to be an individual, inward practice. Even if you meditate in a group setting, you are responsible for being with your own being. No one can do it for you. It's not necessarily easy at first. You actually need to "practice" on a regular basis so that you can help your mind shut off with ease. Eventually, like any other activity or skill, it will start to feel natural and you will "know" how to get to a state of spiritual connection with ease.

Whether you meditate for 5 minutes, 25 minutes, or 50 minutes, you *will* heal yourself. Your authentic connection to your spiritual essence will allow you to move beyond the traumas or pressures of life. Meditating will remind you how big *and* how small you are in this Universe. You will find peace in knowing you are perfect at your core.

Healing your soul is the first step in healing your Earthly life. If you can align with love, then you can work through anything. Distraught peoples around the globe, in every religion, throughout time have found comfort and guidance by taking time for inward focus. Unlike praying, which can sometimes take the form of asking of, or talking to, a higher power; meditation is being present with a cleared mind. No demands, requests, or expectations beyond soulful connection.

This is the point when you might start offering excuses and telling yourself that this is a great theory, but not practical for *you*. You are too busy. Your mind is too active. You have bigger things to worry about than sitting in silence. I hear you. Some days slip by and I miss my meditation. Meditation makes my life easier overall, though, so I always find my way back to my trusty cushions. I don't buy the excuse that your brain is "too busy" and you can't turn it off. If that's the case, you need to meditate even more! People from all walks of life FIND THE TIME to meditate. Rich executives, poor villagers, teen monks, and elementary school children all squeeze it into their day because it makes life better. They want to make the investment of time and focus because they want to live the best life they can…now.

Meditation will wake you up to the life you have. Your changed perspective will impact your decisions, shift your energy, and expand your views. Again, meditation will heal your life by giving you the awareness you need to make the most of your human years. You will crave love, happiness, and abundance in all aspects of your life. You will feel uncomfortable around divisive energy that focuses on scarcity or lack in life. Because you are open to positive, soulful connections, you will attract other people who think, feel, and "walk" through life like you now do. You will start living your life in a state of ease and grace. You will truly live in the flow.

So the title "meditate or die" is a pretty bold statement; sometimes I like being sassy. Obviously we are all going to die physically at some point. There are many ways to look at death and the end of the breathing, human frame; many views are rooted in religious teachings. For the purposes of your meditation practice, religion is a support for your spiritual growth. Religious practice, like meditation, is a way to get a soulful understanding of the human experience. Meditation is a compliment, and never a threat, to any religious affiliation. Going to a house of worship, following a particular set of teachings, and saying prayers to your higher power will not conflict with you sitting in silence, breathing, and focusing on your individual spirit. Learning to quiet the chatter in your mind can only help your religious practice, actually.

Being aware and present in your life, every aspect of your life, is the ongoing gift of meditation. You are alive, awake, aware, and appreciative of your existence. You are not dead; you are alive! You are not unconsciously struggling through your days; you are alive, awake, aware, and appreciative. You meditate so you can stay alive. You meditate so your connection with your heart, your soul, and your passion don't die. You meditate so you *don't* die. You meditate so that you can truly live.

Step 10: Meditate or Die

Let's Get Reflective...

1. What is your experience with meditation?

___

2. How many minutes are you willing to donate to your quiet mindfulness each day? (Beginners: commit to at least one minute per day) ____mins

3. Where do you feel relaxed and peaceful?

___

4. If you're worried about sitting still and meditating, what other activity can you start with that clears your mind? Running, gardening, etc?

_____

_____

_____

_____

_____

Look online or on your phone for a free meditation app. Try it. I'll wait…

5. How was your experience with an app?

_____

_____

_____

_____

_____

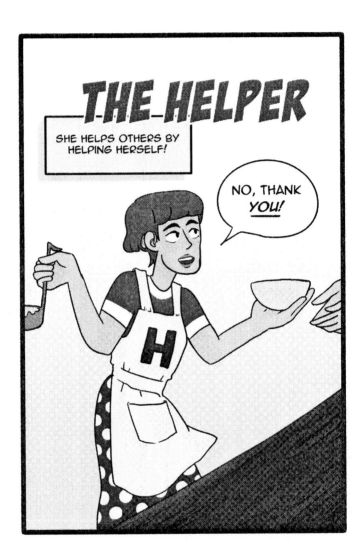

STEP 11

❖

HELP YOURSELF TO HAPPINESS

Women love to give and give and give. We often exhaust ourselves helping others and will even prioritize the comfort of others over our own ease and relaxation. There are distinct pros and cons to this stereotypical female tendency; improve your sense of purpose and value, but you can also wear yourself out. Science has shown that helping others is a key component to boosting your mood; selfless acts get us out of our own drama and stress and provide a fulfilling way to connect with others. The challenge of the modern woman, and maybe all women since the beginning time, is to find the balance between helping others and helping ourselves.

Society makes assumptions about women's

willingness to pitch in and help, whether it's at a school event or a family gathering. There are certain expectations about who will take the lead in volunteer activities and, at the helm, you'll often find a no-nonsense woman. The good news is she is doing something for others that can benefit not only the direct recipients, but also her own emotional health. Giving leads to happiness because you get out of your head and focus on the needs of others. Your world expands to more than just yourself. Furthermore, you join a community that can provide you with support and connections that will benefit you in the future.

That is where you want to be: in a position to help others for their benefit *and* for your benefit. Volunteering your time and energy does not mean that you're sacrificing yourself to the extent that you're a martyr. The goal is to give what you can, but never to give more than you have. In other words, no one wants a burned-out, exhausted helper. Your eventual resentment won't be good for you or those you serve. For the good of everyone involved, decide in advance how much of yourself you have available to help others. Determine if you prefer to do your task alone or if you can only offer yourself if additional supports are available. Make up your mind about how you can be most effective and stick to it. If you go into a "helping" situation with these boundaries, it's more likely that you will enjoy yourself and others will enjoy your presence. The energy flow will be smooth and the interactions will be relaxed. Finally, the mental and emotional rewards will be obvious and you will feel a sense of balance in your life. All good stuff!

Volunteering to lead a meditation class at a local AA center felt great to me in theory and was even better than expected once I started to actually do it. For me, taking time to spend in quiet focus with other like-minded adults was just what I needed to balance out my mostly kid-focused life. When I'm teaching English I'm with children, when I'm home, I'm with children. I am blessed with a short commute to work, but that means I am only kid-free for about four minutes each morning and each afternoon. Leading a class for adults takes some preparation both in regard to the content of the class, but also arranging childcare. I don't mind either task because I enjoy the resulting activity. I do not feel stressed, burdened, or put-out by my volunteering; it's a pleasure for me and the participants. Win-win.

As I've asked you to do before, take stock of what you're already doing and what you'd like to be doing. You have time each day to do a select amount of activities, so only chose those activities that are worthy! Find tasks that balance out your life like adult-only meditation has done for me. Volunteering your time with an interesting organization or doing a task that stretches you in a new direction will not only support those who need it, but will enhance your life. You can choose to add spice to your daily life with volunteering!

Some ladies use volunteering to get a taste of a different world: temporary dog fostering, tutoring students after school, doing hair and nails at a nursing home, leadership on a neighborhood board, babysitting, helping on a horse farm, signing for congregants who are deaf, or refinishing furniture for friends. Volunteering should not be a drag! I had a blast the last time I made hundreds of pancakes for a morning breakfast program. It was super early and the griddle was extremely hot, but it was relaxing to have a rote task to do for 2 hours. I didn't have time to think about anything but what needed to be flipped. Do I want to do that professionally? Nope. I don't even make pancakes at home (husband's domain) and I probably couldn't last much beyond my volunteering shift. Eventually sweating over rows of pancakes would have felt like a drag, and that's when it's time to swap roles. Hand your spatula to another volunteer and take a break. When you're ready, relieve someone else from her duty and enjoy the experience while it lasts.

This all aligns with your marching orders to be a full-time model and to escape from your everyday routine. You may find a love interest while volunteering as well which would assimilate our horny and orgasmic goals in there as well. You never know! When you blow some shit up in your life and live a little bigger, you welcome a host of new opportunities into your realm. By helping others, you are allowing your ego to chill while you enter a selfless state that replicates meditation. I was definitely in a meditative state while supervising all of my pancakes!

So stick your neck out. Start listening for conversations about volunteering gigs. Invent your own project or just offer your services for free to folks you know could benefit. Give yourself as a gift; and set your intentions on happiness and generosity. If you don't feel like your first or second or third attempts are an ideal fit, don't give up. Setting your intentions to be of service is key. Having clear intentions is critical. Eventually you'll find the right way to help others *and* be happy.

Be of service with a loving heart.

Find joy in being generous.

Allow your light to shine and your to soul grow.

Step 11: Help Yourself to Happiness

Let's Get Reflective...

1. Do you already volunteer on a regular basis?
   YES   NO

2. Do you enjoy your current gig(s)? YES NO

3. What do you like to do? (cook, knit, swim, read, paint, run, hold babies)
   - _____
   - _____
   - _____
   - _____

4. How could you take something you enjoying doing and share it with others?

___

5. Where could you look for volunteer opportunities that already exist in your community? (church, library, schools, rec center, shelter, nursing home, police/fire department, hospital)
-
-
-
-

6. When could you make yourself available to help others?

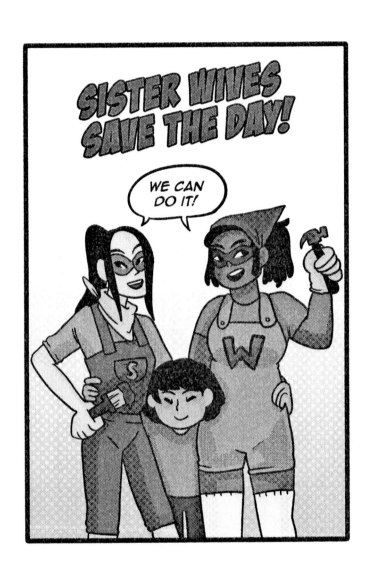

STEP 12

❖

FIND A SISTER WIFE

Mothers are determined to be strong. There must be some conditioning from a young age that tells us a part of our role as a parent is to be a strategic, fierce protector. We are the guardian of our home, our spouse, and our kiddos. We want our children to be secure and we welcome the idea of being the one who keeps danger away. Thank goodness! This common mothering tendency has kept children safe and snug since the beginning of human existence. It's a burden we bear with pride and exhaustion; it takes a lot of energy to be vigilant on a daily basis!

The exhaustive role of Momma-in-charge is precisely why women in every culture, since the rise of communal living, have worked together to raise the children, prepare the food, and tend to the home. Women relying on other women is not a new or novel concept; it's old and normal and necessary. Working together is an efficient concept in any arena, but in mothering it can make the difference in the lives of all participants. Yes, women need help with work, house, and children, but they also need the combined wisdom, grace, and humor that fellow peers provide even more than the logistical support.

Allowing other mothers to "mother" you is a healing process that cannot be underestimated. When you allow another woman to nurture your growth as an adult, you give yourself permission to evolve as an individual. Therefore, as a mother, you're not only supporting your children's growth, you're modeling the learning process for them through your own ongoing evolution.

The easiest way for this type of personal development to transpire is by inviting women into your own home. Allowing another woman to enter your home and be in your space as an equal is pretty awesome. On the spectrum of things necessary for life fulfillment it goes like this: you *want* a massage, you *need* a hot shower, but your soul *desires* the benefits of a sister-wife.

I love referring to the women in my life who co-parent with me in a fluid way as my "sister wives." They love me and they love my children. I know that when they come to my house they are going to stay for hours. We will cook together, supervise the children's activities together, and we will clean together. I am not hosting them or serving them. We are a team and we look for ways to help each other. Upon arrival, bags of food are carried in by children who burst forth from the car or minivan parked out front. Her children instantly mix with my children and they all become a blur of energy buzzing around the house until we demand they go play outside. We are all excited to be together. These visits feed everyone's soul and on some level we understand that this relationship is one important component of our overall happiness.

This level of intimacy between women is equivalent to a part-time spouse. Working together is a way for us to show our love for one another, but we are only able to do this if we allow ourselves to accept help. As a modern woman, self-sufficiency can become a default assumption. We don't need to ask for help because we can do it all. Everyone is working hard so we have to as well. Right?

I want to scream a big "NO!" to this subconscious assertion. I definitely *need* help and I *want* to return the favor. As a mom, I get sick of cooking and disciplining. It is so fun to have someone who is also sick of it, but is totally down for co-creating a great day with me and my brood. Making dinner is not a chore, but a social endeavor that we both do with joy and gossip as we go. Kids run around, but it seems we've both decided not to get stressed about it. They're kids and they're all acting like kids. It's fun to watch each other not lose our temper. If things do get too heated, it's also great for us to tag team the issue.

Necessary Warning: allowing another woman into your house to help you care for your kids, show you how to spice up your favorite dish or load your dishwasher requires a heavy dose of humility. If you hold onto the need to change every poopy diaper or prepare impressive meals instead of accepting the help that is offered, you miss two opportunities.

The first opportunity is to feel efficient; you will get more done with an extra set of hands (if you let them help). So keep on cooking while your friend lets the dog out. Keep chatting while your friend refills the drinks. Don't stop what you're doing to take over every task so that your friend sits like a lump on the couch. Make your time together fun *and* productive.

The second opportunity is your own learning. I have learned how to clean with vinegar, cook a whole meal with one skillet, and make healing tea from women who have let me into their kitchens or taken over mine. Refrain from making everything the way you "always" make it, and stay open to the suggestions of your friend. Try a new flavor combination or cooking style; you may love the results!

If growing and expanding your circle sounds appealing to you, the first step is to set your intentions. Open yourself up to invitations from friends and family members who may want to temporarily co-parent with you. Not everyone will be an easy fit. Sometimes it takes years to cultivate a level of comfort where you can spend hours together or root around each other's refrigerator.

You start where you are and build on the trust you develop over time. At first you may meet at a playground. Next time (months later) you may go on a walk/picnic around a nearby lake. Eventually you will invite her over to your house for lunch on a lazy Saturday. This type of courting is a slow process that yields a deeper relationship. You don't have to talk with her every day. Or even every week! Maybe you get together once a month or every six weeks. Having several different friends means more, and varied, sister wives along the way. There is no need for constant companionship if that doesn't fit your personality or lifestyle.

At some point you'll look around and realize how many genuine relationships you've cultivated with other women. You'll find yourself turning to different women for specific counsel on sensitive topics. Weekends are sprinkled with their visits and you look forward to the different minivans in your driveway. You mother them when they're not mothering you. You hug their kids and she feeds yours. Smiles happen way more than shouting or tears. It's pretty great.

I'm all for girl power. I love being a strong woman. We all agree that women are capable of doing an endless list of things without much outside help. So yeah, you *can* do it all alone, but you probably won't do it very well. You *can* be independent, but your family will be so much stronger if you learn to be interdependent. Why not have a fun support system that makes life better?

Growth is unavoidable when you're open to learning from others. Woman love to help each other and it's great to be on the receiving end, too. There are dynamic women everywhere, probably many ladies you already know would appreciate more adult interaction instead of being home alone with all the little ones.

If you have room in your heart and time in your schedule, it may be time to start dating around.

Who could be one of your future sister wives?

Step 12: Find a Sister Wife

Let's Get Reflective...

1. **Think of a few things you've learned from other women, just by being in their presence or watching them:**

   _____

   _____

   _____

   _____

   _____

2. **List at least 4 women you would like to hang out with more often:**

   ⇒ _____

   ⇒ _____

   ⇒ _____

   ⇒ _____

3. **Are you comfortable having people over to your house?   YES   NO**

4. Are you comfortable hanging out in other people's homes? YES   NO

5. Invite a female friend or family member over for visit or plan a combined trip. Just see how it goes.

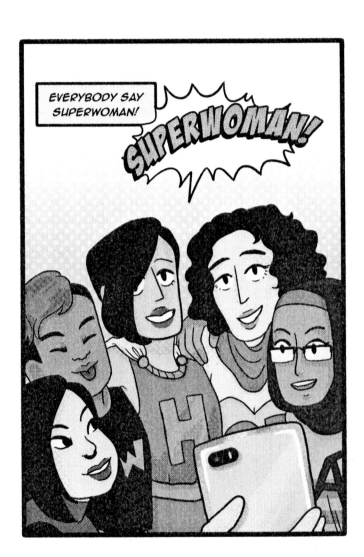

STEP 13

❖

CHOOSE YOUR TRIBE

Growing up in my house, alongside three younger brothers, I learned what kind of people would support my personal development. We were always very honest with each other. Harsh and critical would probably be a better description. As the leader of the (kid) pack, I was the most demanding and oppressive. I wanted things done my way: we needed to play the game I invented, watch the movie I loved (*Can't Buy Me Love*) every night, and settle disagreements in the way I thought was fair. Being the leader of three younger siblings meant making choices, which I was happy to do. I was also willing to impose those choices on others. It worked out great.

Psychologists and common sense agree: our childhood experiences often impact our adulthood. We want to replicate the feelings that gave us joy and comfort while also avoiding certain dynamics we didn't enjoy. One of the gifts of an idyllic childhood like mine is you can focus more on what you want to copy in your grown-up world instead of actively trying to sidestep toxic habits you developed in your youth.

My parents were loving, attentive and always around, but my brothers and I were often left to our own resources when it came to playing and fighting. We had a sense of how far we were willing to take a daring game or a wrestling match. Invariably lines were crossed and bruises were accumulated, but we gained a ton of insight about human interactions in the process. I learned to disagree, debate, and even fight from my brothers. Even though I could force them to do my bidding to a certain extent, it was much easier if I could convince them that they actually wanted to do whatever I was asking of them. Our youthful problem-solving and negotiating was constant. By that, I mean we were always arguing, discussing, or reviewing what was up for analysis.

I still feel like talking it out is the *only* way to work through a problem. I get pretty disoriented when people (including my dear husband) need processing time. He refuses to participate in my "say everything we think now and we'll figure it out together!" game plan. He endures my endless monologues and has to be fairly irritated before he blurts out any unguarded thoughts. But, oh how I love those outbursts! I get to hear what he really thinks, even if it hurts my feelings. My brothers and I still speak without much filter and it feels natural and good.

Without any purposeful effort, I have since surrounded myself with friends who are extremely blunt, frank, and candid. It's nice to always know what people are thinking, even if it's shocking to hear at first. My "sister wives" are tough sometimes, but I can relax in knowing that I will always get the truth from them. Even when it's hard to hear, they steer me away from yelling at my kids, cooking with minimal seasoning, and negative self-talk. My mother was another one of my early trainers; she taught me how to receive open feedback even when I really, really didn't want to listen at all.

In the end, I want us all to have blunt, loving conversations about the things that are important: family, sex, marriage, career, travel, raising kids, and finding space for self-care. We are responsible for choosing our traveling companions on this life journey. We get to decide who we are going to keep and who we are going to gently let go of as we move forward.

As I type this, I'm sitting on the back porch of a log house in Pennsylvania. I am looking at the early sun shimmering on the pond just beyond the back yard. Inside the house my parents, my husband, my three brothers, their spouses, and five little children are all still sleeping. We make an effort to come together twice each year: at Christmas and each summer. We travel from New York, Florida, Colorado, Pennsylvania, and Maryland to whatever spot we choose for our gatherings. We have decided to keep each other as life companions in the midst of busy jobs, bustling offspring, and world travel. Our time together is a constant chatter of silly banter interrupted by serious reflection and debate. We drink beer and cocktails, then hydrate in between. We play yard games. Everyone makes a special dinner on their designated night. We go on exhausting excursions to the beach, kayaking, hiking, or shopping. It's wonderful.

These types of ritual gatherings are important to have in your life. They give your life, and your children's lives, depth and substance. Traditions are beautiful for so many reasons, but they don't have to be created with your extended family. You can nurture your connections with select family members, close friends, and even special neighbors. Your tribe is yours to choose; they are the people in your life who hold your highest admiration and who, in turn, encourage your dreams.

Keep them close, continue to grow through conversations like we have started here, and have confidence to own your unique awesomeness. We are meant to be 100% ourselves. So live a little bigger, enjoy your choices a little more, love with passion (and orgasms), take time to meditate and relax, and never apologize for being completely you.

Chapter 13: Choose Your Tribe

Let's Get Reflective...

1. **Recount at least one time when your group of friends, family, or even neighbors or work colleagues provided support for you in a meaningful way:**

   _____

   _____

   _____

   _____

   _____

2. **Who's in your tribe so far?**

   o _____
   o _____
   o _____
   o _____
   o _____
   o _____
   o _____
   o _____

3. **How do they support your excellence and contribute to your identity?**

_____

_____

_____

_____

_____

4. **What role do you play in your tribe? Describe how your presence brings people together and strengthens connections between individuals.**

_____

_____

_____

_____

_____

THE (SUPER) PEOPLE WHO MADE THIS BOOK POSSIBLE

❖

The funny thing about being married to Brian Brooks is that he'll never tell you what to do...even if you really, really want him to! My husband has consistently supported every decision that I've ever made. I've often questioned his judgment when I was proposing something ridiculous, but he has always maintained that only I know best what I need to be happy. What an amazing gift and responsibility he has given me! He has created the space for me to be the independent woman my parents always hoped I would be. Brian has been my super sexy sidekick for almost two decades and he gets tons of credit for cultivating an unreasonable sense of confidence in me. He also gave me the genetic awesome-sauce to create three wild and wonderful boys.

To Alonzo, you are the epitome of a leader. I watch you assess situations and trust your gut in every arena you are placed. You're headed for greatness and I'm so excited to watch you pursue every ambition with gusto. My Malcolm is efficient and strategic; two of my all-time favorite attributes in a person. You have the style and smarts to make yourself a Brooks on the rise. I'm anxiously awaiting to see your world-wide impact. Sweet Kai, you have a sense of life's purpose: to live in the present moment with love and passion. When I watch you make choices that energize others and yourself, I know that you are the manifestation of the concept, "third times a charm."

To my original tribe: Mom, Dad, Denny, Greg, and Andy, I make myself want to throw up when I think about how much I unconditionally love you. There is no turning off the connection I feel despite our time apart or the miles between us. My prayer is that I can parent as well as Denny and Susie so that my three boys grow up to be as beautiful as my grown-ass little brothers. I'll keep you posted on their progress, but so far, so good.

There are SO many women who have believed in me, encouraged this conversation, and given me feedback on the 13 steps. Jenni (and Lisa!) watered the seed in my soul that said, "you are a writer" and continued to cheer me on with lots of exclamation points and loving emoticons. Carrington and Misti will always be my first coaches who listened, challenged, and steered me along this new and scary path. On the flip side, Meghan, my friend from the way back (virgin club, anyone?) will always be my first client who wanted what I was offering before I even knew what that meant. Ashanti, my beloved, demands that I act as a warrior in all things. Her fierce confidence in me has definitely rubbed off over the years (thank Goddess!) and I am now at peace growing old with her. Heather, my Blow Some Shit Up co-conspirator, you and I dared to daydream and hold each other accountable. Yikes, watch out! Rachel Anne, I cannot believe how much you believed in me. Thank you for reading through the second draft of this book and giving me your take on every nuance…in the most loving way humanly possible. Elizabeth, without your candid insight I don't think I would have been as determined to speak out about the joys of a healthy marriage. Your marriage and our friendship has been a guiding light at all the right times. Susan, I have learned so much about standards and loyalty and friendship from you. You are one smart, fun, super-woman. Bounty, you really know how to love me and I only hope I can make you proud. Thank you for being my #1 Sister-Wife in raising these righteous young men for over a decade. Michelle P, Maru, and Rocky, you ladies showed up right at the point when I wasn't sure what my next steps should be and cheered me across the finish line. I wish your magic on every woman in the world.

And Abe…The Illustrator! You took my ideas and made them exist in a visual realm that I could never have imagined. Your excellence in all things made this process so fun that I dreaded the end of this project. Good problems all around.

ABOUT THE AUTHOR

❖

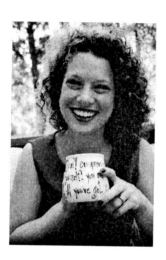

Amy Brooks is an author, teacher and wellness-fanatic who strives to create a safe space for women to prioritize their happiness. She knows that given time and permission, most women will enthusiastically reflect on their life in a loving way.

She renews her peace and her energy on a daily basis in her Maryland home that she shares with three silly sons, two snuggly cats, and one sensational husband.

Join the ongoing conversations at:
AmyBrooksHealth.com

Facebook: *Amy Brooks Health & Wellness Coach*
Stuff Your (Super) Mom Forgot to Tell You

Instagram: *amybrookshealth*

Twitter: *@amybrookshealth*